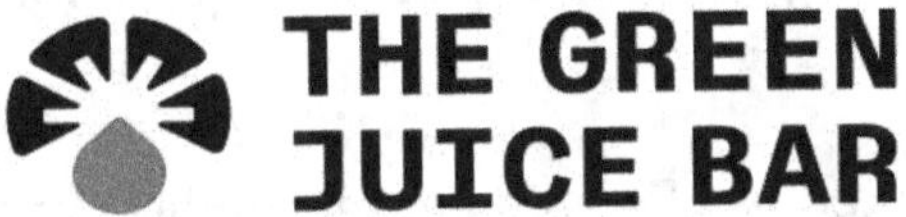

3-Day Organic Juice Cleanse and Fasting Guide

To health, healing, and wholeness… I'll drink to that.

Bridgett N. Green

Printed in the United States of America.

First printing, 2026.
Published by
His Lighthouse Publishing Co. | Atlanta, GA
Email: hislighthousepublishing@outlook.com

Dedication

To God:

Thank You for entrusting me with the vision, strategy, and blueprint to bring The Green Juice Bar from a dream into reality. Every step of this journey is evidence of your guidance, grace, and faithfulness.

In loving memory of my mother, Yvonne Green:

Thank you for planting in me a deep love for food, flavor, and the joy of cooking. Your influence lives in every recipe, creation, and every act of service through this work.

Medical Disclaimer

This guide is shared in the spirit of faith, stewardship of the body, and personal testimony. The information provided in *The Green Juice Bar 3-Day Organic Juice Cleanse & Fasting Guide* is based on personal experience and general wellness practices and is not intended as medical advice, diagnosis, or treatment.

The author and The Green Juice Bar are not medical professionals. This guide is not a substitute for professional medical care. Always seek the counsel of a qualified healthcare provider before beginning any cleanse, fast, or making dietary changes; especially, if you are pregnant, nursing, have a medical condition, or are taking prescribed medications.

Table of Contents

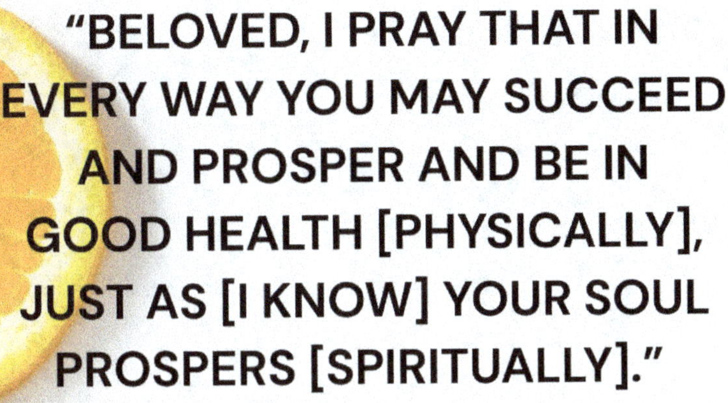
"BELOVED, I PRAY THAT IN EVERY WAY YOU MAY SUCCEED AND PROSPER AND BE IN GOOD HEALTH [PHYSICALLY], JUST AS [I KNOW] YOUR SOUL PROSPERS [SPIRITUALLY]."

3 JOHN 1:2 (AMP)

About The Author

Bridgett Nicole Green is the founder and CEO of **The Green Juice Bar**, a wellness brand rooted in faith, healing, and the transformative power of God's food. Guided by her love for nourishing cuisine and her unwavering belief that food can restore the body, Bridgett stepped boldly into entrepreneurship with a mission to make organic juicing and clean eating accessible to her community.

In 2024, following God's direction, she opened The Green Juice Bar with a clear purpose: to serve fresh, organic juices, smoothies, and meals that support whole-body wellness. Through education, encouragement, and authentic connection, Bridgett has empowered countless customers to reclaim their health and embrace a lifestyle centered on natural, nutrient-rich foods.

Her passion is deeply personal. After being diagnosed with an incurable autoimmune disease, Bridgett confronted the impact of her own eating habits and made a life-altering commitment to change. By eliminating most meats, prioritizing organic fruits and vegetables, increasing physical activity, and standing firmly in her faith, she experienced a complete transformation. In 2022, she was fully healed and released from all medications; a testimony that fuels her mission today.

Now thriving in Mint Hill, North Carolina, Bridgett is a mother, grandmother, best-selling author, entrepreneur, Deacon at Have Life Church, and the driving force behind The Green Juice Bar brand. She is living her purpose with intention: to inspire and guide others toward healing through organic juicing, clean eating, and honoring the body with the foods God created.

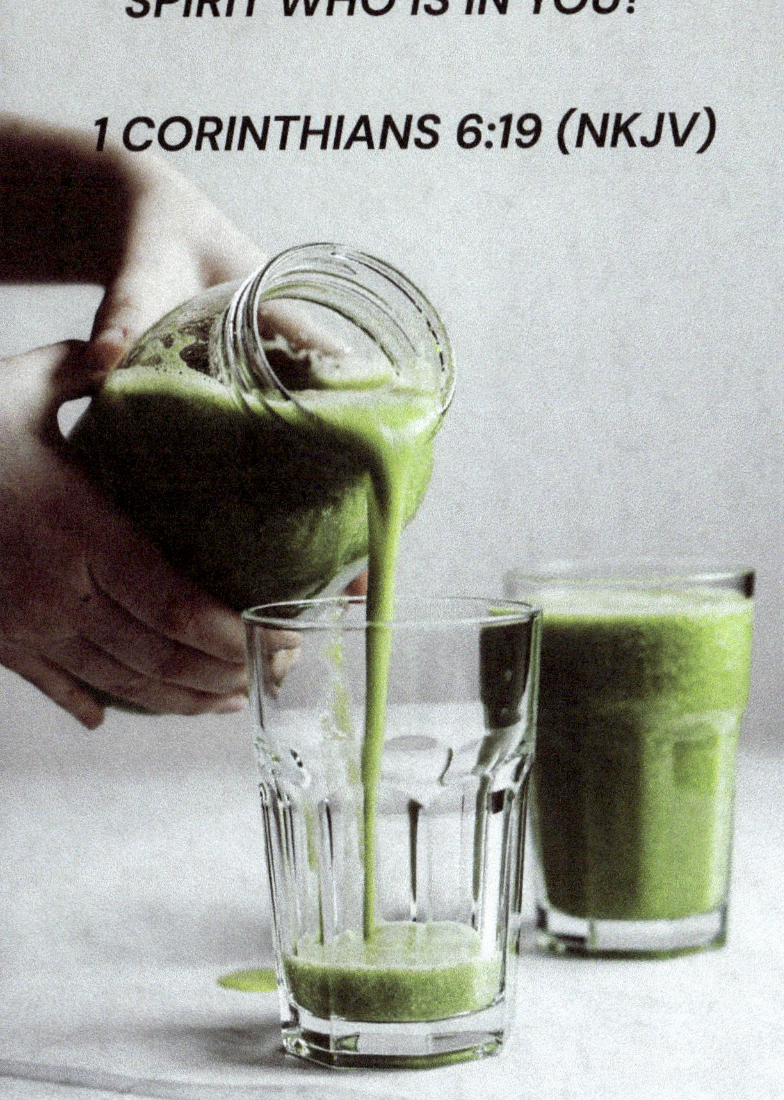

"DO YOU NOT KNOW THAT YOUR BODY IS THE TEMPLE OF THE HOLY SPIRIT WHO IS IN YOU?"

1 CORINTHIANS 6:19 (NKJV)

Introduction

Welcome to The Green Juice Bar Organic Juice Cleanse and Fasting Guide:

We are truly honored that you've chosen to begin this 3-Day Organic Juice Cleanse. Your decision reflects a powerful commitment to restoring your body from the effects of processed foods, excess sugars, toxins, and stress. As you enter this journey, say goodbye to bloating, sluggishness, and imbalance; and say hello to alignment and restoration through organic juicing. This cleanse is an invitation to slow down, turn down our plates and nourish our body, mind and spirit with God's spiritual and natural food.

At The Green Juice Bar, we believe wellness is more than a physical journey; it is a spiritual one. This 3-Day Organic Juice Cleanse and Fasting Guide was created out of obedience, prayer and a commitment to honoring the body as a sacred vessel. Scripture reminds us that our bodies are temples, entrusted to us for stewardship, care, and renewal.

> *"Do you not know that your body is the temple of the Holy Spirit who is in you?"*
> *1 Corinthians 6:19 (NKJV)*

As I reflect on my journey and why the Lord nudged me to write this guide, I believe my testimony will help others to incorporate organic juicing into their diets and implement fasting as a spiritual discipline. These lifestyle changes transformed my physical and spiritual health, ultimately leading to a miracle—the manifestation of healing in my body.

As you read this guide, you will learn the importance of organic juicing, the benefits of completing this three-day juice cleanse, and the undeniable power of fasting.

At the Green Juice Bar, we take pride in using the best organic ingredients during the juicing process. You may question whether organic fruits and vegetables are really necessary and worth the additional expense. I believe so as they are proven to be powerful and more effective. For instance, cold-pressed organic juices allow the body to receive nourishment in its purest form, as God intended. They provide living nutrients that support the body while creating space for stillness, reflection, and spiritual clarity. As the digestive system rests, the body begins repairing and renewing. In this sacred pause, many experience heightened awareness, mental clarity, and a deeper sensitivity to God's voice.

Fasting is both a biblical principle and practice, rooted in God's Word and expressed through humility and obedience. Pairing the three-day juice cleanse with fasting creates space for stillness, reflection, and spiritual clarity. With intentional prayer, fasting shifts to a divine exchange with God. As you drink these organic juices from the Green Juice Bar, may they serve as fuel for your body and a reminder to remain rooted in God, prayer, and gratitude.

Why Organic Matters?

Prior to being diagnosed with an incurable auto-immune disease, I did not fully understand what it meant to honor my body through my food choices. I often chose what was convenient, with no real awareness of the importance of eating healthy or organic foods. During my healing journey, I was encouraged to eat clean meals and incorporate more organic produce into my diet. According to the Cleveland Clinic's 2024 article, *"Organic Foods: Are they better for you?"*, registered dietician Maxine Smith, RD, LD explains that eating organic foods reduces exposure to pesticides while increasing vitamin, mineral, and antioxidant levels. Pesticides are widely used in traditional farming, and cumulative exposure has been linked to many chronic health conditions. However, in the organic farming industry most synthetic pesticides are prohibited and rely primarily on naturally derived pest-control methods, such as plant-based oils, soaps, and minerals that must meet strict safety and environmental standards.[i] Choosing to pursue true health instead of settling for convenience became a defining shift for me, and it's the very reason I commit to using organic fruits and vegetables—not only in my own diet, but also as the standard at The Green Juice Bar.

What is the difference between a Juice Cleanse and a Fast?

The primary purpose of an organic juice cleanse is to gently detoxify the body while resetting the digestive system. During a cleanse, the body is flooded with essential vitamins, minerals, and antioxidants. As the body takes in concentrated vitamins and minerals, toxins are eliminated, which supports weight loss and mental clarity.

How long should I do a juice cleanse? The duration of a juice cleanse may vary from 1 to 7 days but is not suggested for long-term use. This guide's focus is on a three-day organic juice cleanse.

Fasting is the practice of abstaining from food, which generally includes consuming only water or other liquids. While there are several types of fasts, the primary purpose is for deep detoxification or spiritual discipline. The duration of a fast may vary and often includes intermittent hours, days, or weeks. This guide's focus is on the biblical practice and principle of fasting. Before deciding to complete a juice cleanse or fast, please consult your healthcare provider.

Why Choose The Green Juice Bar's 3-Day Organic Juice Cleanse or Fast?

Not all juice cleanses are created equally. The Green Juice Bar's 3-Day Juice Cleanse was designed with you in mind; all organic cold-pressed juices, free of added sugars, preservatives, and harmful pesticides. Cold pressed juicing retains more vitamins, nutrients, and antioxidants compared to store-bought juice cleanses and was designed to support liquid fasting.

The Green Juice Bar's 3-Day Organic Juice Cleanse provides maximum benefits, whether you are completing the cleanse or pairing it with a fast; each resulting in restoration, transformation, and mental clarity.

Who is This Cleanse and/or Fast For?

Whether you're looking to kickstart a healthier lifestyle, lose weight or get spiritually aligned, this cleanse and/or fast is for you. It's suitable for both beginners and those who regularly consecrate. If you have any underlying health conditions, we recommend that you consult a healthcare professional before starting.

In the following pages, you'll find everything you need to successfully complete your 3-day cleanse and/or fast, including step-by-step guidance and tips for a smooth experience.

This cleanse is an invitation:

- To release what no longer serves you.
- To quiet distractions.
- To realign your mind, body and spirit

As you begin this journey, listen closely, pray often, and trust that God is working in both seen and unseen ways; bringing health, healing, and wholeness from the inside out.

To health, healing, and wholeness... I'll drink to that

---

[i] Tudi, Muyesaier et al. "Agriculture Development, Pesticide Application and Its Impact on the Environment." International journal of environmental research and public health vol. 18,3 1112. 27 Jan. 2021, doi:10.3390/ijerph18031112

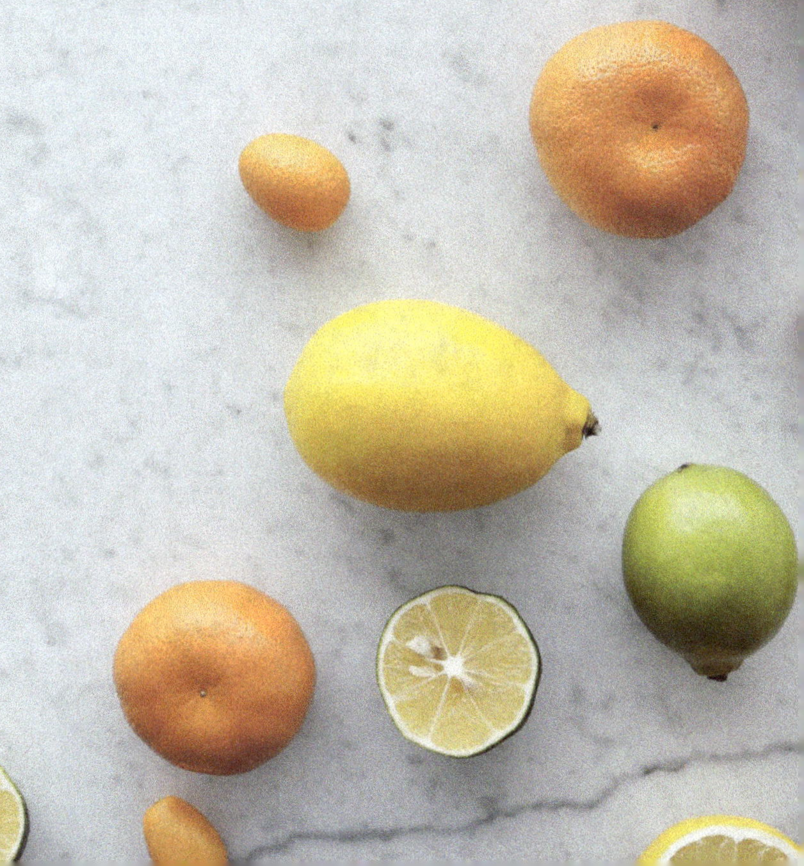

"BLESSED ARE THOSE WHO HUNGER AND THIRST FOR RIGHTEOUSNESS, FOR THEY SHALL BE SATISFIED."

MATTHEW 5:6 (NASB1995)

Benefits of an Organic Cold-Pressed Juice Cleanse

When you incorporate an organic cold-pressed juice cleanse into your wellness routine it is a physical and a spiritual act of honoring the body God entrusted to you. By choosing foods grown from the earth, untouched, unaltered, and full of life, you are selecting the food God intended from the beginning.

"Then God said, "I give you every seed-bearing plant on the face of the whole earth and every tree that has fruit with

seed in it. They will be yours for food."
Genesis 1:29 (NIV)

Organic cold-pressed juices also preserve the fullness of God's provision through natural sources of vitamins, minerals, enzymes, and living nutrients, which allows your body to receive them in the purest form.

When I completed my first juice cleanse, I wasn't sure what to expect. I immediately noticed how I felt and looked upon completion. I felt lighter, my skin was glowing, and I experienced an improvement in my wellbeing. The overall benefits are numerous but here are a few, each aligned with scripture and biblical principles of health, stewardship, and wholeness.

1. Strengthens Immunity

Organic cold-pressed juices are rich in vitamin C, antioxidants, and plant-based nutrients that help strengthen your immune system and fight off illness. Ingredients like citrus and ginger help support immune health.

God provides natural tools to support healing — and organic juices are among them.

"And their fruit will be for food and
their leaves for healing."
Ezekiel 47:12 (NASB1995)

2. Improves Digestion & Gut Health

Organic juices contain living enzymes that support digestion and gut balance. Papaya, pineapple, celery, cucumber, and leafy greens help reduce bloating and improve gut health. God's food is purposeful, powerful, and designed to support the body He created.

"He provides food for those who fear
him; he remembers his covenant forever.
He has shown his people the power
of his works."
Psalm 111:5–6 (NIV)

3. Increases Natural Energy

Organic cold-pressed juices offer a clean, natural, sustained energy source without caffeine or artificial stimulants. Apples, pineapples, oranges, and berries provide natural sugars, antioxidants, and enzymes that aid in digestion and provide a midday boost of energy. Leafy Greens and beets help oxygenate the blood while providing long-lasting energy, stamina, and endurance. God strengthens us spiritually — and He provides natural foods that strengthen us physically.

> *"...Shall renew their strength; They shall mount up with wings like eagles, They shall run and not be weary, They shall walk and not faint."*
> *Isaiah 40:31 (NKJV)*

4. Supports Detoxification

Your body is wonderfully designed by God to detox on its own. Organic cold-pressed juices simply support and accelerate this natural process. Celery, cucumber, and papaya naturally flush toxins from your body, while lemon supports and maintains liver function. Just as God removes what does not belong spiritually, He provides foods that help remove what does not belong physically.

*"I will sprinkle clean water on you, and
you will be clean; I will cleanse you from
all your impurities and
from all your idols."*
Ezekiel 36:25 (NIV)

5. Promotes Radiant Skin

Vitamin-rich juices nourish the skin from within. Carrots, citrus, cucumber, beets, ginger, spinach, kale, pineapple, watermelon, berries, and papaya help reduce inflammation and acne, boost collagen production, improve circulation, and hydrate the skin. God's food renews us from the inside out.

*"He satisfies your mouth with good
things, so that your youth is renewed
like the eagle's."*
Psalm 103:5 (NKJV)

6. Aids in Healthy Weight Management

Organic juices help curb food cravings, balance blood sugar levels, and promote a sense of fullness. Replacing processed foods with God-made ingredients supports a healthy metabolism. Healthy choices help break unhealthy cycles.

"It is not good to eat much honey..."
Proverbs 25:27 (NKJV)

7. Reduces Inflammation & Supports Joint Health

Ginger, lemon, pineapple, and leafy greens contain powerful anti-inflammatory compounds that reduce joint pain and swelling. God cares about the health of your bones, joints, and entire body.

"Pleasant words are like a honeycomb,
Sweet and delightful to the soul and
healing to the body."
Proverbs 16:24 (AMP)

8. Hydrates & Replenishes Electrolytes

Cold-pressed juices hydrate the body while providing essential electrolytes and minerals that support circulation and overall function. Just as your spirit thirsts for God, your body thrives when it receives pure, life-giving hydration.

"My soul thirsts for God,
for the living God."
Psalm 42:2 (NKJV)

To health, healing, and wholeness... I'll drink to that.

"SO WHETHER YOU EAT OR DRINK OR WHATEVER YOU DO, DO IT FOR THE GLORY OF GOD."

1 CORINTHIANS 10:31 (NIV)

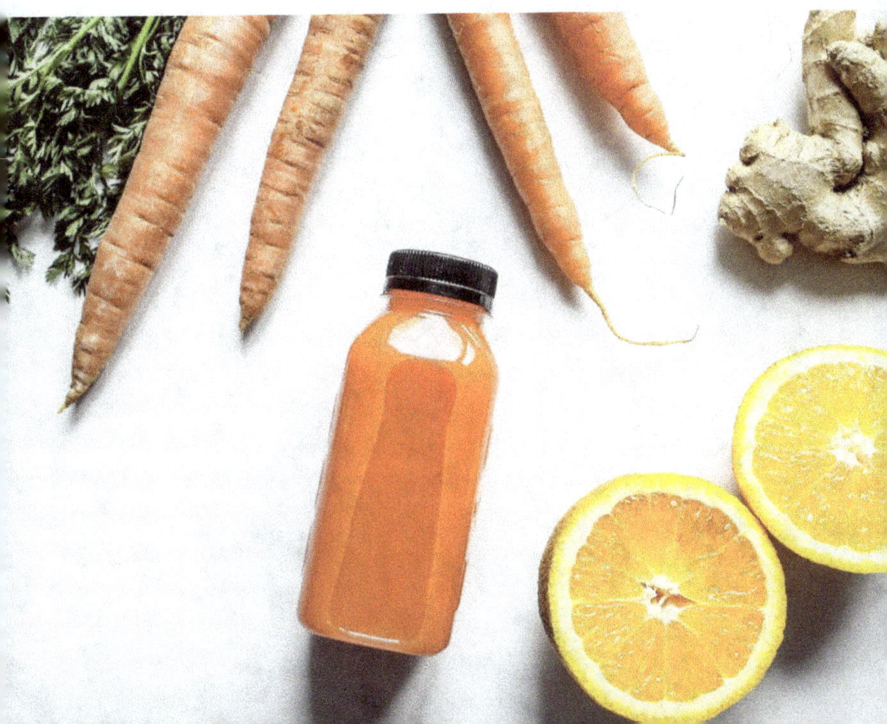

The Power of Organic Juicing

Organic juicing is one of the most powerful and underrated nutritional decisions you can implement. Studies show when fresh fruits and vegetables are juiced, their nutrients become highly concentrated, offering the body a powerful supply of vitamins, minerals, and antioxidants. Choosing organic ingredients guarantees that what you put into your body offers true nourishment without the burden of unwanted chemical exposure.

"So whether you eat or drink or whatever you do, do it for the glory of God."
1 Corinthians 10:31 (NIV)

Most organic produce is grown without synthetic pesticides, herbicides, or chemical fertilizers. This is important because everything in or on the produce is passed during the juicing process. By choosing organic juice, you lower your risk of toxin exposure and support the natural systems God designed to keep you healthy and whole.

"Beloved, I pray that in every way you may succeed and prosper and be in good health [physically], just as [I know] your soul prospers [spiritually]."
3 John 1:2 (AMP)

Cold-pressed organic juices also preserve living enzymes and phytonutrients that strengthen your digestion, immunity, and cellular renewal. These nutrients are absorbed quickly, allowing the body to be nourished while the digestive system rests. This is a vital component of cleansing and fasting.

Additionally, organic juices gently support the body's natural detox pathways, especially within the liver, kidneys, and intestines.

Autophagy begins, which is the body's built-in process of cellular renewal. This detoxification works in harmony with the body's natural rhythm, bringing clarity, balance, and renewal from the inside out.

Lastly, organic juicing aligns perfectly with the biblical principle of fasting. During times of consecration, the body, mind, and spirit are nourished spiritually and physically. Through the word of God, prayer, and organic juicing the whole person is being nourished and aligned with God's voice.

"Man shall not live by bread alone, but by every word that proceeds from the mouth of God."
Matthew 4:4 (NKJV)

At The Green Juice Bar, organic juicing reflects a commitment of integrity, purity, and care. We believe in honoring the body as a sacred vessel while providing support to maintain a healthy lifestyle.

"Don't you realize that your body is the temple of the Holy Spirit, who lives in you and was given to you by God?"
— 1 Corinthians 6:19 (NLT)

To health, healing, and wholeness... I'll drink to that.

Beyond Detox: The Spiritual & Physical Renewal of a Juice Cleanse

A juice cleanse does more than remove toxins from your body; it is also create intentional space for clarity, alignment, and spiritual sensitivity.

1. Improves Mental Clarity & Focus

Removing processed foods and caffeine is the simplest way to sharpen the mind and reduce brain fog. A renewed mind begins with better choices.

*"..but be transformed by the renewing of
your mind."*
Romans 12:2 (NIV)

2. Promotes Better Sleep

When your body isn't overworked by heavy digestion, it's able to rest more deeply and restore itself. Removing stimulants such as caffeine, sugar, and processed snacks helps create space for peaceful, uninterrupted sleep. Rest is not only restorative, but it is prophetic, sacred, and a true gift from God.

*"I will both lie down in peace, and sleep;
For you alone, O Lord,
make me dwell in safety."*
Psalm 4:8 (NKJV)

3. Encourages Mindful Eating Habits

A cleanse naturally slows your eating rhythm and invites you to become more intentional with every food choice. True wisdom is reflected in how we steward our bodies, especially in the days that follow the juice cleanse.

"Teach us to number our days, that we may gain a heart of wisdom."
Psalm 90:12 (NKJV)

4. Creates a Fresh Start for a Healthy Lifestyle

A cleanse serves as a spiritual and physical reset, making it easier to maintain healthy habits long after the cleanse ends. God specializes in new beginnings including your health journey.

"Behold, I am making all things new."
Revelation 21:5 (NASB1995)

When you choose The Green Juice Bar's organic cold-pressed juice cleanse, you are aligning with God's design for your body, detoxing spiritually and physically while gaining clarity, wisdom, and long-term wellness for your body, mind, and spirit.

"DRAW NEAR TO GOD AND HE WILL DRAW NEAR TO YOU."

JAMES 4:8 (NKJV)

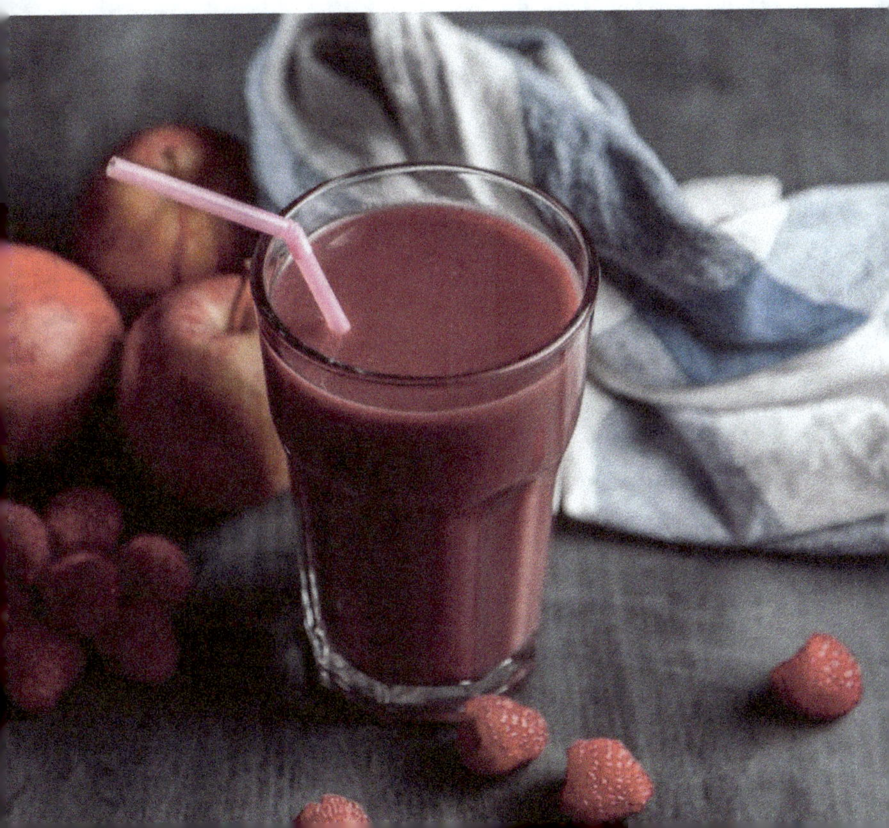

The Power of Fasting

Fasting is one of the most powerful spiritual disciplines. Long before it was recognized for physical benefits, it was established as a divine invitation to pause, listen, and realign your heart with God. Jentezen Franklin, pastor and author of the book *Fasting: Opening the Door to a Deeper, More Intimate, More Powerful Relationship with God*, states that "fasting brings one into a deeper, more intimate and powerful relationship with the Lord."[ii] Fasting, from a spiritual perspective, is not about deprivation; rather, it is about spiritual discipline and devotion to God. It is the intentional setting aside of food and any physical comforts to create space for spiritual intimacy. When the noise of constant consumption is quieted, the spirit becomes more attentive, receptive, and sensitive to God's voice.

> *"Draw near to God and He will draw near to you."*
> James 4:8 (NKJV)

Fasting Creates Spiritual Clarity

One of the first spiritual benefits many experience during fasting is clarity. As the body slows down and distractions lessen, the mind becomes still. This stillness allows room for reflection, prayer, and discernment. Fasting helps quiet the flesh so the spirit (Holy Spirit) can be heard. Spiritual clarity enables better decision-making by prompting us to slow down and listen before taking action. God's voice is easier to recognize—not because He speaks more loudly, but because we are finally listening. This is one of the reasons I fast often. Life can be busy but when I fast I am reminded to slow down, quiet my quiet my environment so I may hear God clearly. In Exodus, Moses received the greatest revelation during a 40-day fast, the Ten Commandments (Exodus 34:27-48).

"Be still, and know that I am God."
Psalm 46:10 (NKJV)

Fasting Cultivates Humility & Dependence on God

Fasting reminds us that our strength does not come from food alone, but from God Himself. It reorients our dependence from self to the Holy Spirit. In moments of hunger or discomfort, fasting teaches surrender, trust, and humility. It is a gentle reminder that God is our source, sustainer, and provider; He is Jehovah Jireh!

"It is written, Man shall not live by bread alone, but by every word that proceeds from the mouth of God."
Matthew 4:4 (NKJV)

Fasting Sharpens Spiritual Sensitivity

When physical appetites are restrained, spiritual sensitivity is heightened. Many people report increased awareness, deeper prayer, and stronger discernment during times of fasting. The spirit becomes more alert, responsive, and aligned. This sensitivity is not emotional, but a spiritual alignment. Fasting tunes the heart and ears to recognize what is from God and what is not.

"My sheep hear My voice, and I know them, and they follow Me."
John 10:27 (NKJV)

Fasting Supports Repentance, Renewal & Inner Healing

Biblically, fasting is often paired with repentance and renewal. It provides space to release burdens, forgive, reflect, and invite God into areas that need healing. As the body rests, the soul is given room to be restored. Fasting allows us to confront what we've been avoiding and surrender it fully to God.

*"Create in me a clean heart, O God,
And renew a right and steadfast spirit
within me."*
Psalm 51:10 (AMP)

Fasting Aligns the Body with the Spirit

Fasting is one of the most powerful tools God gives us to realign every part of who we are to Him: body, soul, and spirit. Each part responds differently, yet they all move toward harmony when we choose to abstain from physical appetites and turn our attention toward God. This alignment produces peace, balance, and discipline that extends beyond the fast itself.

*"Now may the God of peace Himself
sanctify you completely; and may your
whole spirit, soul, and body be preserved
blameless..."*
1 Thessalonians 5:23 (NKJV)

Fasting Prepares the Heart for Transformation

Fasting also creates fertile ground for transformation to occur. It softens the heart, strengthens resolve, and increases obedience. What begins as a temporary act often produces lasting spiritual fruit; such as, greater discipline, deeper faith, and renewed purpose. This 3-day fast is not about perfection but about posture, a willing heart and an open spirit. The ultimate outcome is a surrendered life.

"Turn and come to Me with all your heart [in genuine repentance], With fasting and weeping and mourning [until every barrier is removed and the broken fellowship is restored]."
Joel 2:12 (AMP)

Fasting Activates Breakthrough

Fasting is a duty of every Christian. The Bible explains in Matthew 6 that the duties of every Christian are giving, praying, and fasting.

Pastor Franklin also explains in the same book that when these three practices come together in a believer's life, they create a type of threefold cord that is not easily broken. Fasting paired with prayer and giving has been known to accelerate healing, restoration, and undeniable breakthrough. I have been the recipient of this type of breakthrough in my health, finances and family. Fasting is the catalyst to miraculous breakthrough.

> *"Because of your unbelief; for assuredly, I say to you, if you have faith as a mustard seed, you will say to this mountain, 'Move from here to there,' and it will move; and nothing will be impossible for you. However, this kind does not go out except by prayer and fasting."*
> Matthew 17:20-21 (NKJV)

A Sacred Invitation

This cleanse and fast is an invitation to abide deeply in our Heavenly Father — to release the need to strive but instead rest in His presence. It is a call to listen more closely by embracing stillness and quietness, meditating on His word, and allowing God to restore what has been depleted. As you fast, may your spirit be realigned to God, your faith deepened, and your heart renewed.

Reflection Questions

For Prayerful Consideration

Take time to sit quietly with these questions and journal your responses. During prayer, reflect on them or return to them throughout your fasting journey. Open your heart and allow God to meet you in honesty and truth.

1. What led me to this fast, and what is my heart's intention?
2. What distractions or habits am I being invited to release during this time?
3. What areas of my life do I need greater clarity, direction, and/or peace?

4. What emotions or thoughts have surfaced as my body and mind have slowed?
5. Is there anything God is revealing that requires surrender, forgiveness, or trust?
6. What does health, healing, and wholeness look like for me in this season?

[ii]Franklin, Jentezen. *Fasting: Opening the Door to a Deeper, More Intimate, More Powerful Relationship with God.* Lake Mary, FL: Charisma House, 2007.

"YOUR BODY IS HIS TEMPLE. YOUR HEALING IS HIS PROMISE. YOUR JOURNEY STARTS NOW."

BRIDGETT N GREEN
AUTHOR & CEO OF THE GREEN JUICE BAR

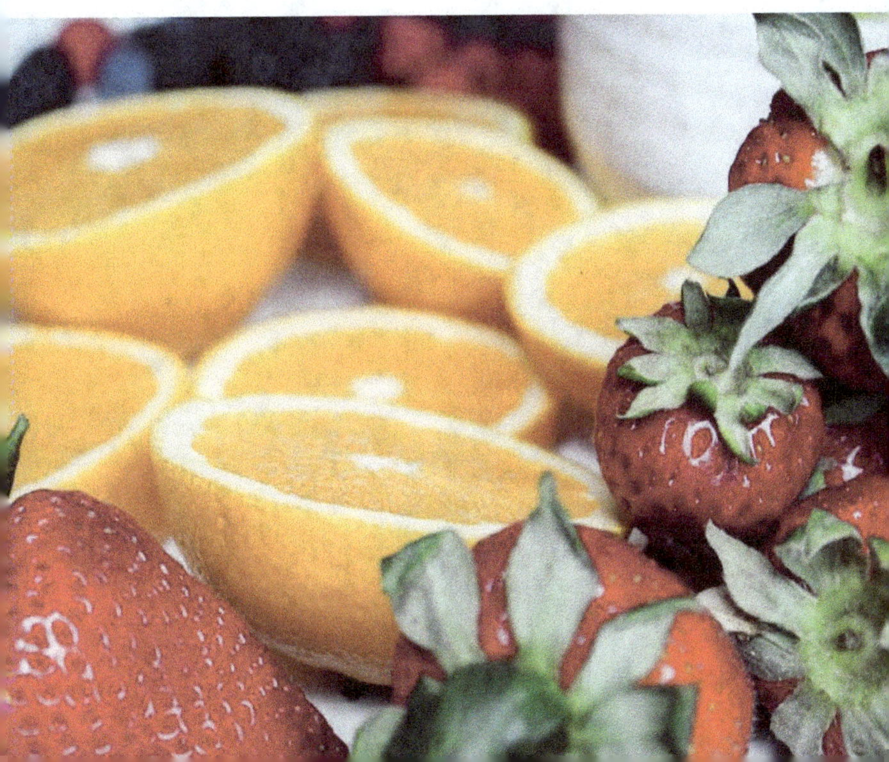

Preparing for the Cleanse or Fast

How to Properly Plan for the Organic Juice Cleanse or Fast

A successful organic juice cleanse or fast requires more than just drinking juice—it's about preparing your body, choosing the right juices, and easing back into regular meals in a way that maximizes benefits. Here's a step-by-step guide to ensure a smooth and effective cleanse.

Set Your Goals

Before starting, identify your reason for cleansing or fasting. Are you looking to boost energy, improve digestion, reduce bloating, or reset from unhealthy eating habits? Are you seeking spiritual alignment or guidance? Defining your goals will help you stay motivated throughout this journey.

Prepare Your Body (Pre-Cleanse/Fast Phase)

To lessen detox symptoms, I highly suggest you begin making dietary changes 3 to 5 days before starting.

- Increase: Intake of fresh fruits, vegetables, whole grains, nuts, and water.
- Reduce: Caffeine, alcohol, sugar, dairy, processed foods, and red meat.
- Eliminate: Fried foods, refined sugars, and artificial additives.

This transition helps your body adjust and makes the overall experience smoother.

Stay Hydrated

While juicing, remember to drink extra water to help flush toxins from your body. Aim for at least 8-10 glasses of water daily. Drinking herbal teas, coconut water or warm lemon water will also support digestion and hydration.

Listen to Your Body

It's normal to feel lightheaded or experience mild headaches as your body detoxifies. If you feel extremely fatigued, try:

- Sipping herbal tea or coconut water for extra electrolytes.
- Resting and avoiding intense workouts.
- Consuming a handful of raw nuts or avocado, if absolutely necessary.

Transition Back to Solid Foods (Post-Cleanse/Fast Phase)

After your cleanse or fast, reintroduce solid foods gradually to avoid shocking your digestive system. Follow a post-cleanse diet for at least 2-3 days:

- **Day 1:** Fresh fruits, smoothies, light salads, steamed vegetables.

- **Day 2:** Whole grains, lean proteins, and nuts.
- **Day 3:** Gradually reintroduce dairy, legumes, and cooked foods.

Note: Avoid jumping straight into heavy or processed foods, as this can cause bloating and discomfort.

Maintain a Healthy Lifestyle

This juice cleanse isn't just a one-time detox—it's an opportunity to reset your eating habits. After completing the cleanse or fast, continue incorporating organic cold-pressed juices, whole foods, and hydration into your daily routine to sustain the benefits. This is important to maintain the results.

By following this structured approach, your juice cleanse or fast will be more effective, enjoyable, and beneficial for long-term wellness.

'INTERMITTENT FASTING IMPROVES THE BODY'S DEFENSES AGAINST OXIDATIVE STRESS AND INFLAMMATION, THE CORNERSTONES OF AGING AND DISEASE."

MARK MATTSON, PHD
NEUROSCIENTIST, JOHN HOPKINS

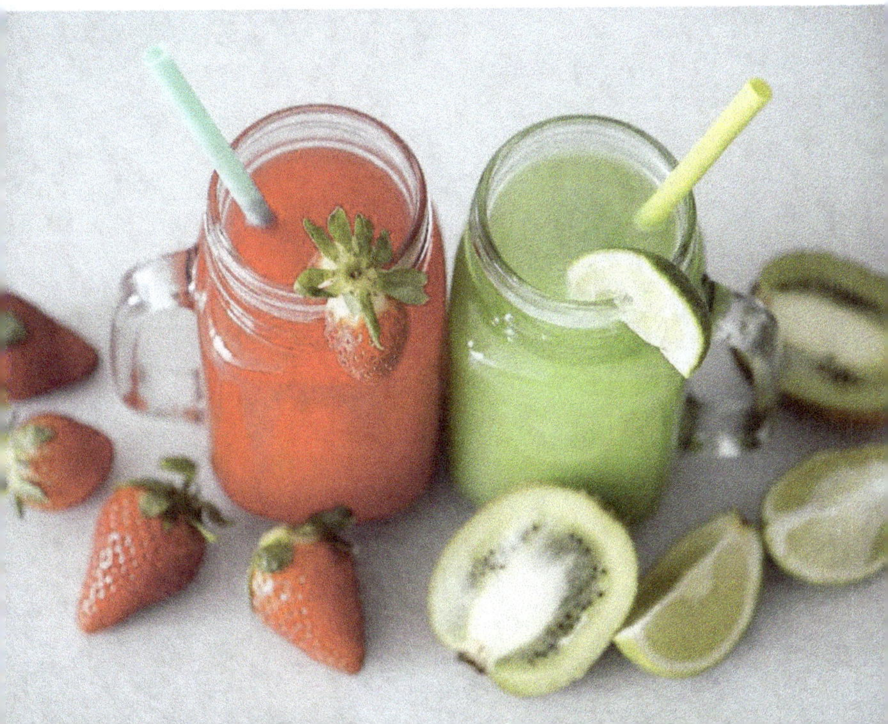

The 3-Day Organic Juice Plan

How It Works

During this 3-day cleanse, you'll consume a series of seven organic cold-pressed juices from the Green Juice Bar daily. Each will be consumed every 2-3 hours and are carefully curated to provide essential nutrients, antioxidants, and hydration to support your body's natural detoxification process. The cleanse may be used during a fast, as a meal replacement, or to supplement a healthy meal plan. The daily juice drinking schedule example is based on my personal experience and additional research. However, feel free to alter it based on your needs and/or preference.

Drinking water during the juice cleanse is highly recommended. Water is essential for staying hydrated and aids in the detoxification process. Drink Up and Enjoy!

Daily Juice Drinking Schedule Example:

1. Morning (7am): Berry Beet Fusion (Heart, Cholesterol & Blood Sugar Health)
2. Mid-Morning (10am): The Defender (Vitamin C Boost & Immunity Support)
3. Lunch (12 Noon): Tropical Balance (Energy Boost & Gut Health)
4. Afternoon (2pm): Super Greens (Refreshing & Hydration)
5. Early Evening (5pm): The Defender (Boost Immunity, Supports Digestion, Detox)
6. Night (7pm): Super Greens (Supports Detoxification & Increases Metabolism)
7. Evening Snack (8pm): Berry Beet Fusion (Heart, Cholesterol & Blood Sugar Health)

Note: The juice drinking schedule is a suggestion only. Please adjust as needed. Drinking water during the juice cleanse is highly recommended.

By following this cleanse, you'll nourish your body, reset your digestion, and emerge feeling lighter, clearer, and more energized.

Guided Fasting Prayer

A Daily Prayer for Alignment & Renewal

Here is a prayer you may use to start your fast. Find a quiet space. Take a few deep breaths, breathing in through your nose and exhaling through your mouth. Allow your body to settle and your mind to become focused on our Heavenly Father.

Prayer

Heavenly Father,

I come before You with humility and gratitude. I thank You for being Yahweh, Lord Jehova, the true and living God (1 Thessalonians 1:9). I praise You for who You are; You are my Lord and Savior (Acts 16:31). Lord, You are an everlasting God and the creator of the all the earth (Isaiah 40:28). I am grateful that You are all-knowing, all-seeing and all-powerful

(Psalms 139). I love, trust and adore You. I exalt in Your name and praise You Lord with all of my heart; I will tell of all the marvelous things You have done (Psalm 9:1). Great is Your faithfulness.

Father, I invite You into this time of consecration. I fully surrender my desires, will, and appetite to You. As I set aside physical comforts to draw closer to You, open my ears to hear you, my eyes to see, and my heart to receive from You.

I am grateful for this time of fasting and intimacy with You. As I rest in You, quiet my mind and increase my sensitivity to Your voice. As distractions fall away, increase my focus and sharpen my discernment. As hunger arises, grant me the strength to endure and remind me that You are my source and sustainer.

Father, search my heart and reveal anything that needs healing, correction, or release. Create in me a clean heart and renew a steadfast spirit within me (Psalms 51:10). I surrender completely to You and invite Your peace that transcends all understanding (Philippians 4:7). I invite Your guidance as I abide in you (Psalms 25:4). And I welcome Your strength to fill every part of me (Isaiah 41:10).

Guide me through this fast with grace. Let this time produce lasting fruit: greater discipline, clarity, and renewed alignment with Your will.

In Jesus' name, Amen.

Daily Scripture References & Declarations for Fasting

Day 1 – Humility, Surrender & Preparation

Fasting begins with surrender—laying aside control and inviting God to lead. These scriptures anchor the heart in humility and readiness.

"Turn to Me with all your heart, with
fasting, with weeping,
and with mourning.
Joel 2:12 (NKJV)

Bridgett N. Green

"Humble yourselves in the sight of the Lord, and He will lift you up."
James 4:10 (NKJV)

"Lay aside every weight, and the sin which so easily ensnares us."
Hebrews 12:1 (NKJV)

Today's Declarations

- Today, I humble myself before the Lord.
- I release every weight, distraction, and unhealthy attachment.
- I surrender my will, my appetite, and my expectations to God.
- I choose obedience over comfort and faith over control.
- As I fast, my heart softens, my spirit opens, and my focus clears.
- God is lifting me, guiding me, and preparing me for renewal.
- Today, I am surrendered.
- Today, I am attentive.
- Today, I begin this fast with trust and humility.

Day 2 – Renewal, Strength & Clarity

As the fast continues, God renews strength and sharpens spiritual awareness. These scriptures encourage perseverance and transformation.

"But those who wait on the Lord shall renew their strength."
Isaiah 40:31 (NKJV)

"Do not be conformed to this world, but be transformed by the renewing of your mind."
Romans 12:2 (NKJV)

"My grace is sufficient for you, for My strength is made perfect in weakness."
2 Corinthians 12:9 (NKJV)

Today's Declarations

- Today, I receive renewed strength from the Lord.
- My body is sustained, my mind is clear, and my spirit is alert.

- God's grace is sufficient for me in every moment of this fast.
- I reject fatigue, doubt, and distractions.
- I embrace clarity, endurance, and spiritual focus.
- My mind is being renewed, and my heart is aligned with God's will.
- Today, I walk in strength.
- Today, I walk in clarity.
- Today, I remain faithful and focused.

Day 3 – Restoration, Breakthrough & Alignment

The final day of fasting is often marked by restoration, peace, and alignment. These scriptures seal the work God has begun.

"He restores my soul; He leads me in the paths of righteousness."
Psalm 23:3 (NKJV)

"Now may the God of peace Himself sanctify you completely."
1 Thessalonians 5:23 (NKJV)

"Draw near to God and He will draw near to you."
James 4:8 (NKJV)

Today's Declarations

- Today, I receive restoration—spirit, soul, and body.
- What God has begun in me is being completed with peace and purpose.
- My body is aligned, my spirit is renewed, and my heart is anchored in truth.

- I carry forward discipline, wisdom, and gratitude.
- This fast has strengthened my faith and sharpened my discernment.
- I move forward whole, restored, and aligned with God's design.
- Today, I am restored.
- Today, I am aligned.
- Today, I walk forward in wholeness.

Closing Affirmation

- The Word of God sustains me.
- His presence strengthens me.
- His peace rests upon me.

How to Break Your Fast

A Gentle Return to Nourishment

Breaking your fast is just as important as beginning it. After days of rest, prayer, and intentional nourishment, your body is receptive, sensitive, and ready to be reintroduced to whole foods with care. This moment is an extension of your fast—an opportunity to honor the work God has done within you.

Begin Slowly

Start with foods that are easy to digest and as close to their natural form as possible. Allow your body to awaken gradually.

Recommended first foods:

- Fresh fruit (such as berries, melon, apple, or pear)
- Steamed vegetables (zucchini, carrots, spinach, or squash)
- Light soups or broths
- Smoothies made with whole fruits and vegetables

Be mindful of what you consume and how it makes you feel.

Avoid Immediately After the Cleanse

For the first 24 hours, continue to avoid foods that can overwhelm the digestive system:

- Fried or greasy foods
- Heavy meats
- Dairy products
- Refined sugars and processed foods

- Excess caffeine or alcohol

Choosing restraint now helps preserve the benefits of your cleanse.

Listen to Your Body

Your body will speak clearly after a fast. Pay attention to how foods make you feel—energized, heavy, clear, or sluggish. Let this awareness guide your choices moving forward.

Cover Your Nourishment in Prayer

Before your first meal, pause and pray:

Prayer of Gratitude

Father God,

Thank You for carrying me through this time of fasting and renewal. I am grateful for what I learned, how I've grown and what I will carry with me after these three days.

As I return to eating, help me to choose foods that honor my body and sustain the work You have begun within me. May I continue in discipline and wisdom. Let every bite I eat nourish my body and be received with thanksgiving.

In Jesus' name, Amen.

Post Cleanse/Fast Meal Plan

1–3 Day Post-Cleanse Meal Plan

Continuing the Work with Wisdom

The days following your cleanse are a sacred continuation of the journey. Your body is reset, your awareness is heightened, and your choices now help preserve the benefits you've gained.

Day 1 – Gentle Reintroduction

Focus: Hydration, simplicity, and digestion

Morning

- Warm lemon water or herbal tea

- Fresh fruit (berries, melon, or apple) or a light smoothie

Midday

- Green juice or vegetable juice
- Steamed vegetables (spinach, zucchini, carrots)
- Light vegetable soup or broth

Evening

- Large salad with leafy greens, cucumber, avocado, lemon, and olive oil
- Optional: a small portion of quinoa or brown rice

Day 2 – Strength & Balance

Focus: Sustained energy and nourishment

Morning

- Smoothie with fruit, greens, and plant-based milk or water
- Handful of nuts or seeds

Midday

- Whole-food bowl (steamed vegetables, quinoa or brown rice, avocado)
- Green juice or fresh-pressed juice

Evening

- Light protein (beans, lentils, chickpeas, or baked tofu)
- Roasted or steamed vegetables

Day 3 – Returning to Rhythm

Focus: Balance, consistency, and sustainability

Morning

- Whole fruit or smoothie
- Herbal tea or water

Midday

- Balanced meal: vegetables, whole grains, and clean protein

- Fresh juice or infused water

Evening

- Home-cooked, whole-food meal
- Emphasis on portion control and mindful eating

Foods to Continue Limiting

- Processed foods
- Refined sugars
- Excess salt
- Fried foods
- Alcohol

Returning to Routine

Carrying the Cleanse Into Everyday Life

As you return to your normal routine, remember that wellness is not found in perfection, but in consistency. This cleanse was never meant to be a moment—it was meant to be a marker. A pause that reoriented your habits, your appetite, and your awareness.

You may not eat perfectly every day—and that's okay. What matters is intention. Choose progress over pressure. Discipline over guilt. Grace over extremes.

Carry Forward what You've Learned

- Listen to your body
- Choose foods that give life
- Create space for prayer and reflection
- Drink water often
- Rest when needed

Let this cleanse/fast be a reminder that you are capable of discipline, renewal, and alignment.

THE SHOPPING LIST

Prepare With Intention

Here is a suggested shopping list for pre- or post-cleanse/fast. Choose organic produce whenever possible, especially for pre- and post- cleanse/fast meal plans.

FRUITS

- APPLES
- LEMONS
- BERRIES
- AVOCADOS

VEGETABLES

- SPINACH
- KALE
- ZUCCHINI
- CARROTS

PROTEIN

- BEANS
- LENTILS
- CHICK PEAS
- TOFU
- CHICKEN
- FISH

GRAINS, SEEDS AND OILS

- BROWN RICE
- QUINOA
- CASHEWS
- ALMONDS
- PUMPKIN SEEDS
- CHIA SEEDS
- OLIVE OIL

BEVERAGES

- ORGANIC COLD-PRESSED JUICE*
- WATER
- COCONUT WATER
- HERBAL TEA

*THE GREEN JUICE BAR

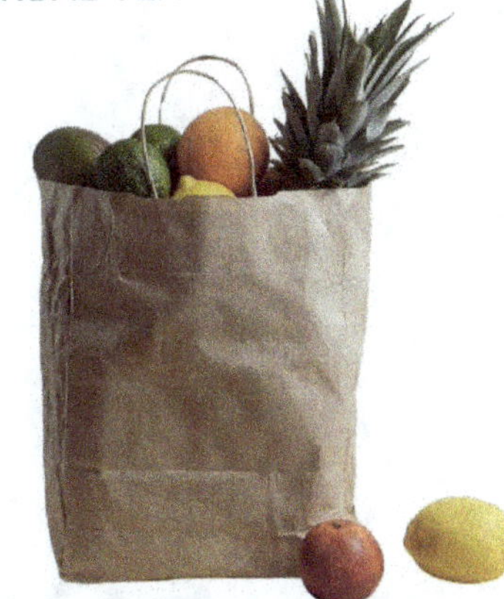

3- DAY CLEANSE & FAST TRACKER

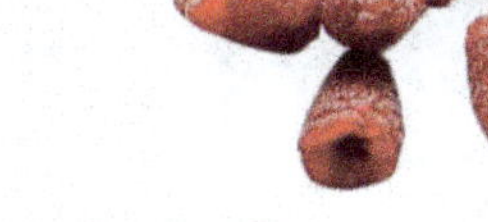

DAY 1 – HUMILITY, SURRENDER & PREPARATION

WHAT SCRIPTURE(S) DID YOU FOCUS ON TODAY?

WHAT DID GOD REVEAL?

HOW MANY JUICES & WATER DID YOU DRINK TODAY?

HOW DO YOU FEEL?

3- DAY CLEANSE & FAST TRACKER

DAY 2 – RENEWAL, STRENGTH & CLARITY

WHAT SCRIPTURE(S) DID YOU FOCUS ON TODAY?

WHAT DID GOD REVEAL?

HOW MANY JUICES & WATER DID YOU DRINK TODAY?

HOW DO YOU FEEL?

3- DAY CLEANSE & FAST TRACKER

DAY 3 – RESTORATION, BREAKTHROUGH & ALIGNMENT

WHAT SCRIPTURE(S) DID YOU FOCUS ON TODAY?

WHAT DID GOD REVEAL?

HOW MANY JUICES & WATER DID YOU DRINK TODAY?

HOW DO YOU FEEL?

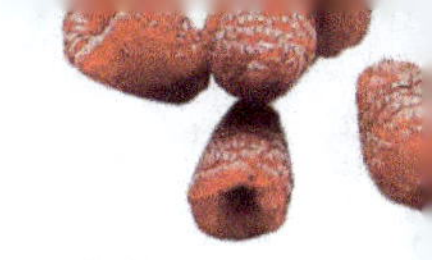

Final Thoughts & Encouragement

Celebrating Your Achievement

Congratulations! You've successfully completed your 3-day organic cold-pressed juice cleanse, and that is something to be incredibly proud of. Cleansing is more than just a reset for the body—it's a commitment to your health, well-being, and self-care. By choosing nourish yourself with pure, organic ingredients, you've taken an important step toward a healthier you.

Incorporating Organic Juicing into Your Lifestyle

Your journey doesn't end here. The benefits of juicing extend far beyond these three days, and I encourage you to continue incorporating organic cold-pressed juices from The Green Juice Bar into your daily routine. Whether it's starting your morning with a revitalizing green juice, adding a nutrient-packed juice as an afternoon pick-me-up, or using fresh juices to complement a balanced diet, your body will thank you for the continued nourishment.

Honoring the Vessel God Has Given You

Your body is a sacred gift, a divine vessel entrusted to you by God. When we choose to fuel ourselves with God's food, we show gratitude for this gift and respect for the life we've been given. Taking care of your health is not just about looking and feeling good—it's about honoring the temple that God has blessed you with.

"Or do you not know that your body is a temple of the Holy Spirit who is in you, whom you have from God, and that you are not your own? For you have been

*bought with a price; therefore glorify
God in your body."
1 Corinthians 6:19-20 (NASB1995)*

Let this cleanse serve as a reminder of your strength, your discipline, and your dedication to your well-being. Continue to make mindful choices that support your health goals and know that each step forward is a step toward a life of healing, wholeness, and abundance.

Thank you for allowing The Green Juice Bar to be a part of your journey. Stay committed to nourishing your body, and may you continue to flourish in health, healing, and wholeness.

With Gratitude & Encouragement,
Bridgett N Green

The Green Juice Bar